HELLO!
This is your
body speaking

PAIN MANAGEMENT

Mary Wheeler, LMT

www.TouchOfMary.com

Second Edition Copyright © 2016 Mary Wheeler, LMT
ISBN: (e)
ISBN: 978-0-692-61426-6 (sc)
Mary Wheeler rev. date 01-04-2016

First Edition Copyright © 2012 Mary Wheeler, LMT
ISBN: 978-1-4525-4888-3 (sc)
ISBN: 978-1-4525-4887-6 (e)
Library of Congress Control Number: 2012905016

The author of this book does not dispense medical advice or prescribe the use of any technique as a form of treatment for physical, emotional, or medical problems without the advice of a physician, either directly or indirectly. The intent of the author is only to offer information of a general nature to help you in your quest for wellbeing. In the event you use any of the information in this book for yourself, which is your constitutional right, the author and the publisher assume no responsibility for your actions.

Cover Illustration by Barbara B Gleason
Illustrations by Barbara B Gleason / BGleason Design & Illustration
Edited by Christine Lorenz, B.A., LMT – Eugene, OR
Authors Photograph by Kelli Hollenbeck / KelliD Photography - Sherwood, OR

Cover design by BliinkDesign.com
Interior design by Catherine Baduin

Contents

Guiding Thoughts...2

Self Evaluation...6

Sitting 13

Standing..22

Walking...32

Lying Down..40

System of Change 46

Acknowledgments...51

Praise for "Hello! This is your body speaking.".................53

About the Author..59

Resources...61

This book is dedicated to all of you who believed in me before I believed in me.

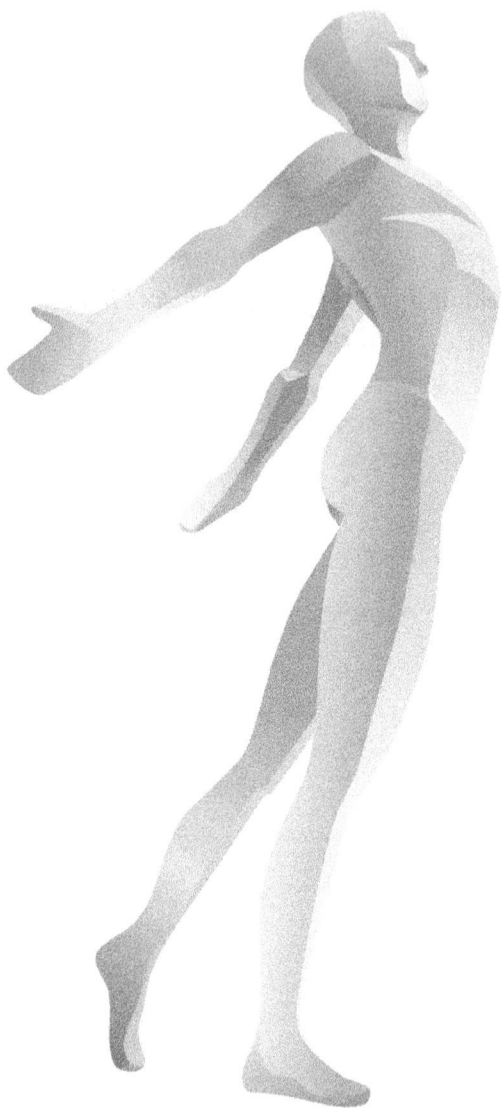

"Life Expresses Itself Through Movement!"
Alain Géhin, D.O.

Take notes about how you feel right now.

_____

_____

_____

_____

_____

_____

_____

_____

Pain Management is: Awareness, Relief, Prevention

_____

_____

_____

_____

_____

_____

_____

*Additional tools at **www.TouchOfMary.com***
We Have Tutorial Videos

Guiding Thoughts

I have been a Massage Therapist since 1993. My main practice is run out of my home and I also work part time seeing an MD's patients at his office. I specialize in movement analysis.

On my way to discovering my own path of self-empowerment, I realized sharing my own process was going to be a big part of that path. Developing the discipline to sit down and write and publish this book was a struggle for me. In the end, the need to share this information pushed me to "just do it." And I had lots of help from my friends.

I work with and teach my clients over many visits. The goal of this book and the videos at TouchOfMary.com is to teach you *(expose you to new information)* without knowing you personally, your physical history of aches, pains or joys --- and without watching you move across the room to access how I can help. So these tools are all about me being able to be "there" with you as you explore you.

I believe that each person's inner self *(self observation and understanding)* knows what is best for that individual. Developing a working relationship with your inner self is where this book intends to lead you, the reader. Taking notes about your own self-observations is immensely helpful! I hope that a small seed is planted by reading these words and that you will cultivate it to help you on your own path of self-empowerment.

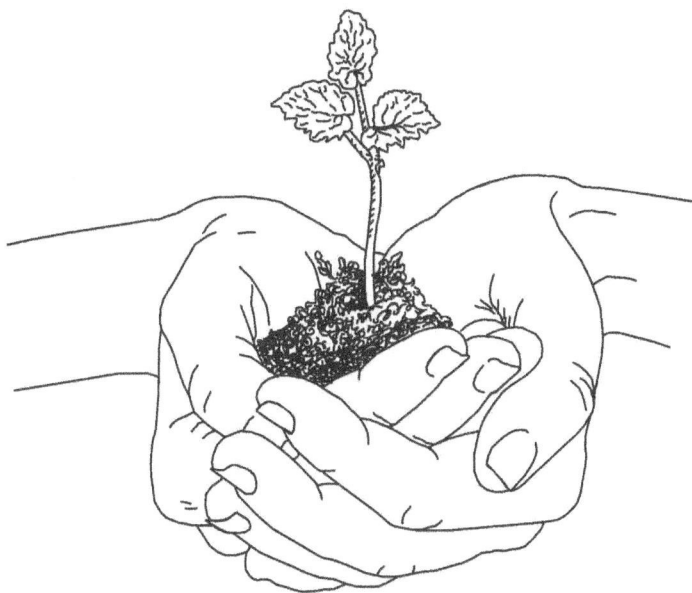

It is important for the stage to be set.

This book is designed as a guide to your own body. After assimilating this book's concepts you can review and work with the separate chapters in any order that you wish. The end result is that you will no longer need this book because you will have the concept working inside of yourself.

> *The ability to observe your own body mechanics objectively is the key to effectively using the information in this book. I have included short phases at the beginning of each chapter to remind you how.*

"Ask, Listen, Respond," is the same as saying "Take Inventory, Evaluate, Make Change," which is the same as "What am I doing? How is this affecting me? What can I do differently?"

If at any time you become confused by any of the content, simply skip ahead to Chapter 6 "System of Change" and read it through for clarity and an overview.

Now it is time for the curtain to lift.

Take notes about what you did for the last two days. Was anything out of the normal for you?

_____

_____

_____

_____

_____

_____

_____

_____

Pain Management is: Awareness, Relief, Prevention

_____

_____

_____

_____

_____

_____

_____

*Additional tools at **www.TouchOfMary.com***
We Have Tutorial Videos

CHAPTER 1

Self Evaluation

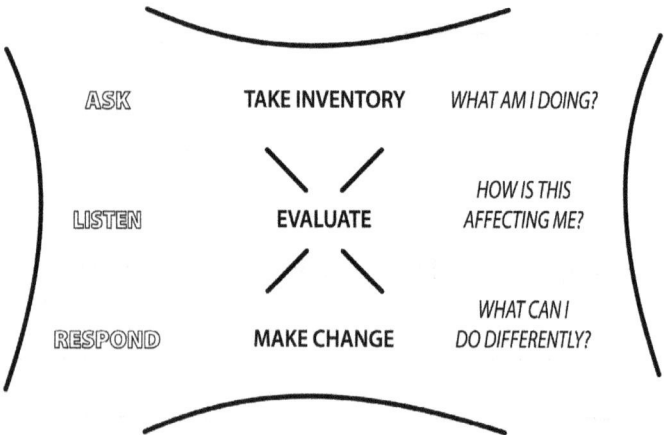

ASK	TAKE INVENTORY	WHAT AM I DOING?
LISTEN	EVALUATE	HOW IS THIS AFFECTING ME?
RESPOND	MAKE CHANGE	WHAT CAN I DO DIFFERENTLY?

Act: as if it is the first time you are taking inventory every time you take inventory!

You: will be open to new information with this approach.

*Additional tools at **www.TouchOfMary.com***

Self Evaluation

I have an inner network that is a communication system within my own body. I believe you have one too. So let's start helping you get to know your inner network.

We all notice the lights at the intersection. Are they red, green or yellow? It's a good system because we all agree on what those lights mean and do what they ask us to do, so we can all drive cars fast and close together on a paved road.

Your body has a similar type of system. I call this system *Be-Friending My Pain.*

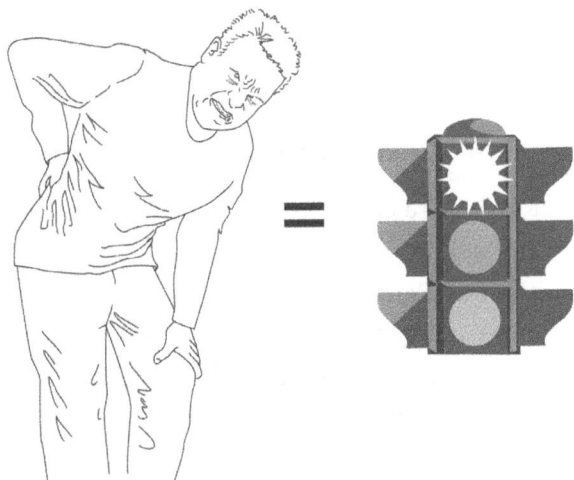

Why be-friend my pain? Because it is the signal light at the intersection.

- Feeling good
- Tired or Hurting
- Pain - When you feel pain it means STOP now!

How many of us stop when it hurts?

It is important to listen to your pain *(whisper or shout)* and then let the pain guide you to new behavior.

Having more joy and pleasure is something all of us want. I believe developing communication with your own body sensation system *(a pleasure/pain feedback loop)* will lead you to a more healthy and happy life.

So where to begin?

Well let's just say you're going to have to be willing to be a little crazy and talk to yourself. In order to evaluate, an inventory has to be taken. In my mind I am the mayor of the city called "my body." (Choose your own metaphor if mine does not work). I have a waste department, water department, electrical department, planning department, management team etc. You get the point here?

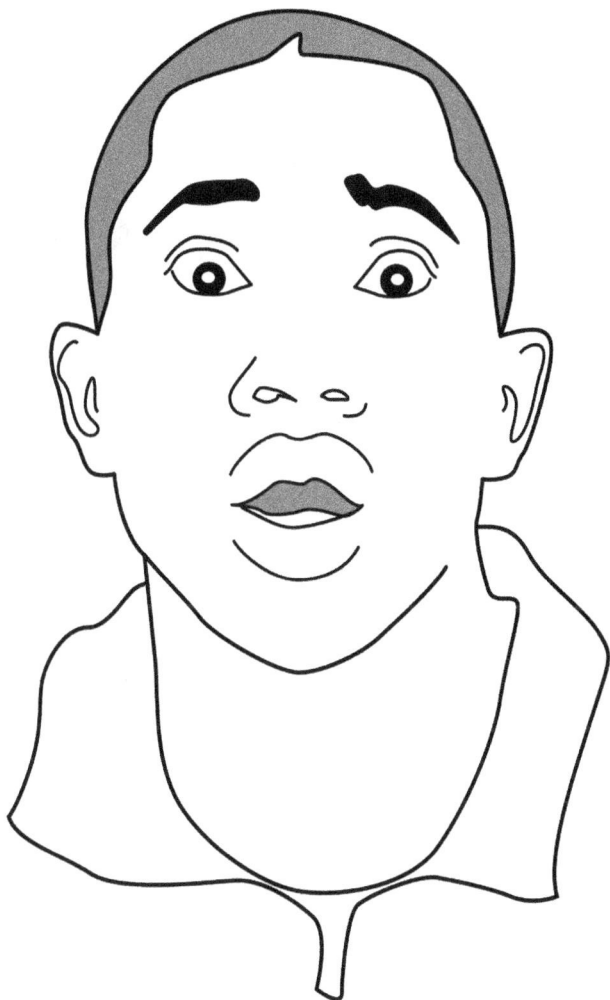

Okay, I am ready if you are.

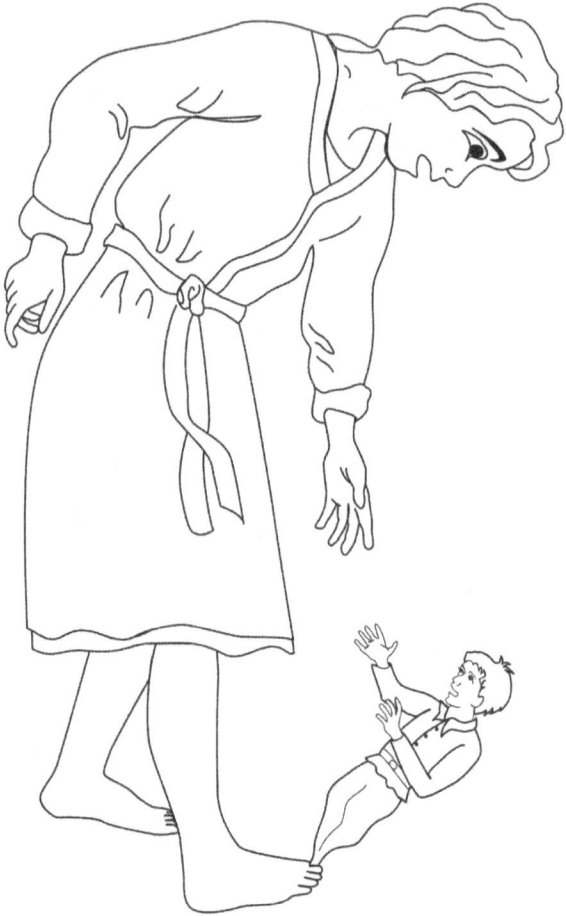

Hello!

Exercise 1:

Get comfortable in a quiet environment.

Breathe in and out several times.

Close your eyes.

Now let your mind scan your body from head to toe and just notice whatever comes to mind.

Now let your mind be pulled to any place in your body (example: Right foot: little toe).

Imagine this body part as a person and introduce yourself to it. *(Play with me here).*

Let your imagination have free reign.

Ask how it (the body part) is doing and if there is any thing you can do for it. Now in your mind give it whatever it has asked for.

When finished ask if it needs anything else right now and follow through by again giving what is asked for. Say "good-bye, nice to meet you, just call if you need anything and I will stop by again."

Take several more breaths and then open your eyes.

You can do this with any body part or body system. Remember to think in metaphors and look at what that part of the body does (example: the small intestine sorts what to absorb and what to discard of the food taken in).

There is no limit to how often you can do this. Even visiting a good feeling body part is relevant. Most of all have fun getting to know your-self in a new and creative way.

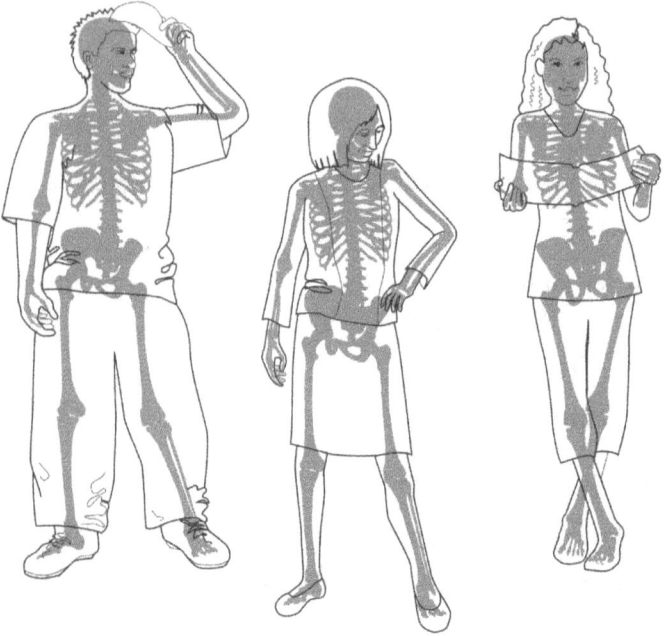

The focus of this book will be on the biomechanics of the body in a very basic way. It is a simple way to build the relationship with / within yourself.

CHAPTER 2

Sitting

ASK   **TAKE INVENTORY**   *WHAT AM I DOING?*

HOW IS THIS
AFFECTING ME?

LISTEN   **EVALUATE**

RESPOND   **MAKE CHANGE**   *WHAT CAN I*
DO DIFFERENTLY?

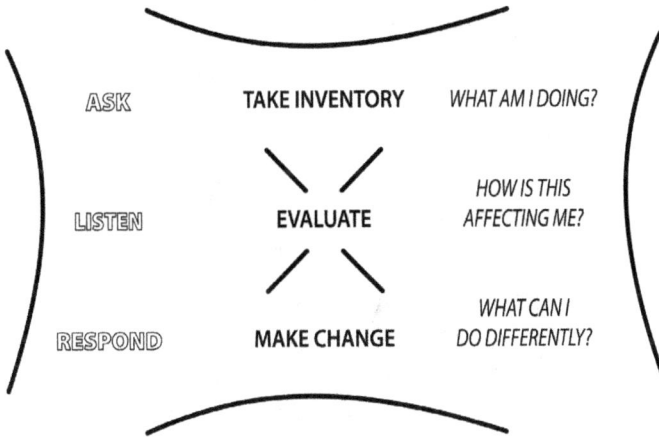

Act: as if it is the first time you are taking inventory every time you take inventory!

You: will be open to new information with this approach.

*Additional tools at **www.TouchOfMary.com***

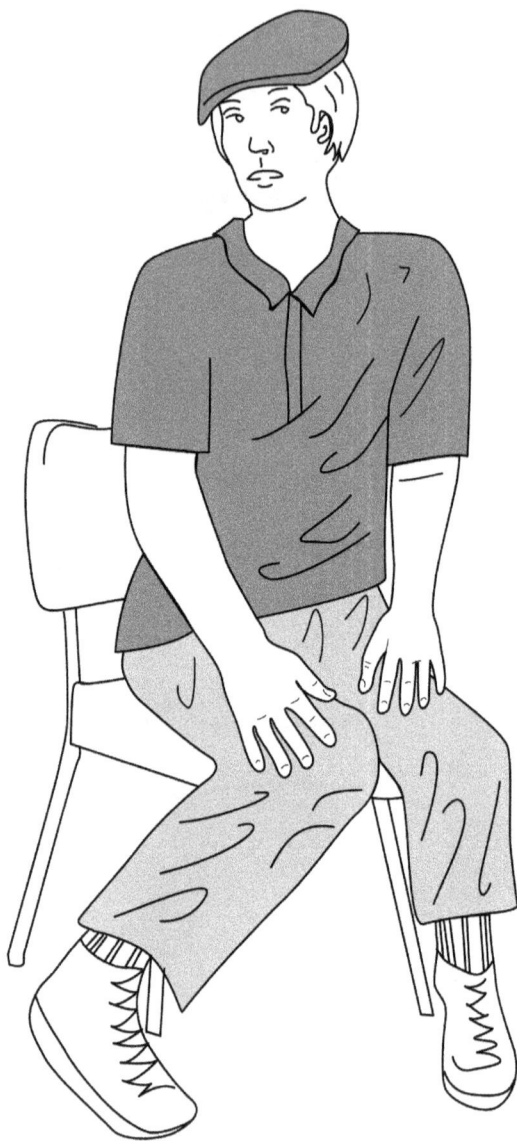

I don't think I can sit here any longer!

Sitting

So to begin with, the body was not made to sit for long periods of time. As a child you fidgeted in a chair and you became uncomfortable. Then you got into trouble (ugh)! So we learn to override the discomfort signals that tell us to move. We don't even hear the pain warning us after a time. The chair is an invention of man that can be very comfortable. Yet we as humans have insisted that the body is going to sit, for hours on end.

So let's look at how we sit. We will use sitting at a computer desk as an example. Then you can *adapt* the information to driving a truck or using a sewing machine.

> *Once you have the general concept and a working dialog with your body, the body will give you feedback if your correction is sufficient.*

Chair

The chair has a firm surface that supports you. If it has armrests, they need to be low enough that when your elbows are bent 90 °your arms will clear the armrest.

The depth of the seat should be no deeper than the length of you thigh.

The back of the chair should be there to meet and support your body.

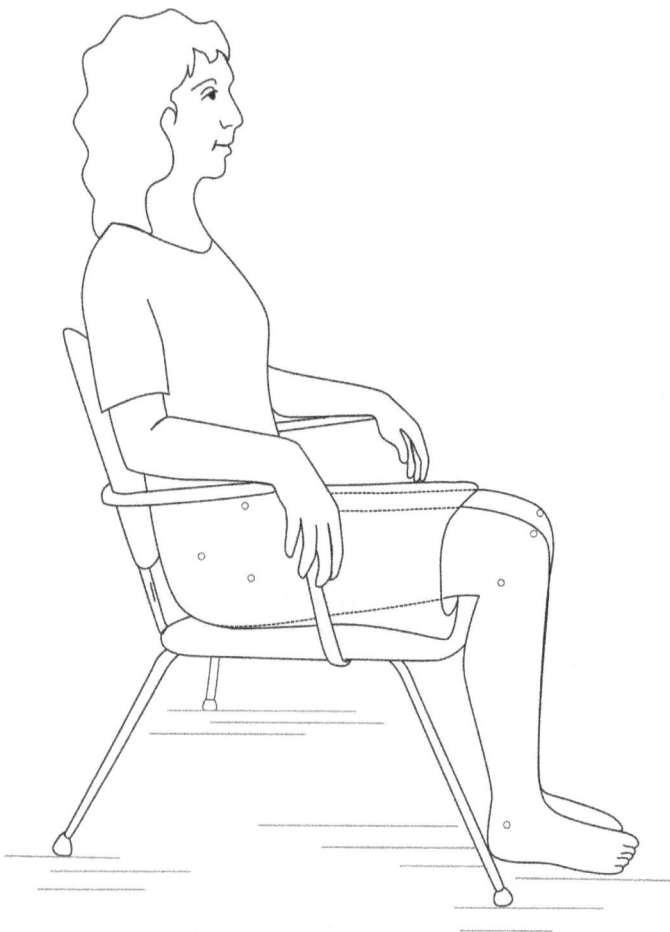

For me this is a comfortable position to sit in. What is a good position for you to sit in?

Finding your position

Sit forward in your chair, feet resting on the floor (or footrest) and arms free of armrests.

Begin leaning back and forth, rocking on the sit bones (the bones you feel when sitting on a hard surface), finding the most central position and coming to rest here. Lengthen the spine and relax the body and it *should* stack up from this central sit bones position with the head balancing on top. Stay here for a bit, just breathing, with your eyes closed. Scan your body and imprint this position in your mind. This is the most supported position to sit in.

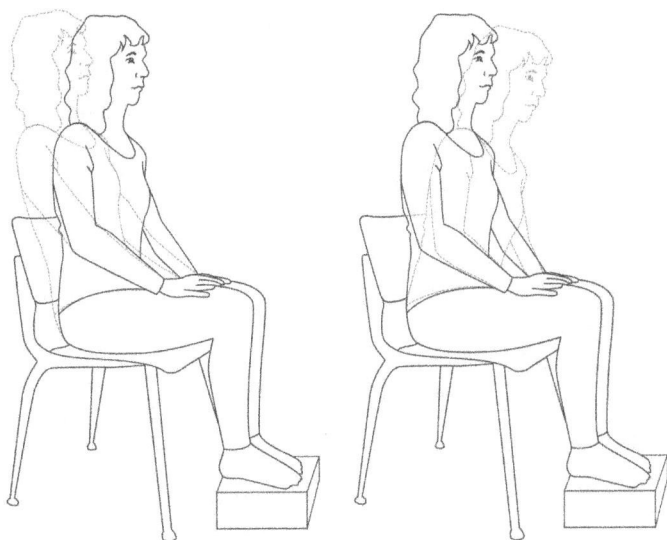

To get yourself squarely between each of your sit bones, push into the floor with one foot at a time feeling what is happening with the pelvis on the chair. When you do this you want to notice how the leg is pulling on the pelvis and where your weight distribution from the upper body is. This can be used throughout the day to check if you are balanced or (if not) readjust so that you are balanced.

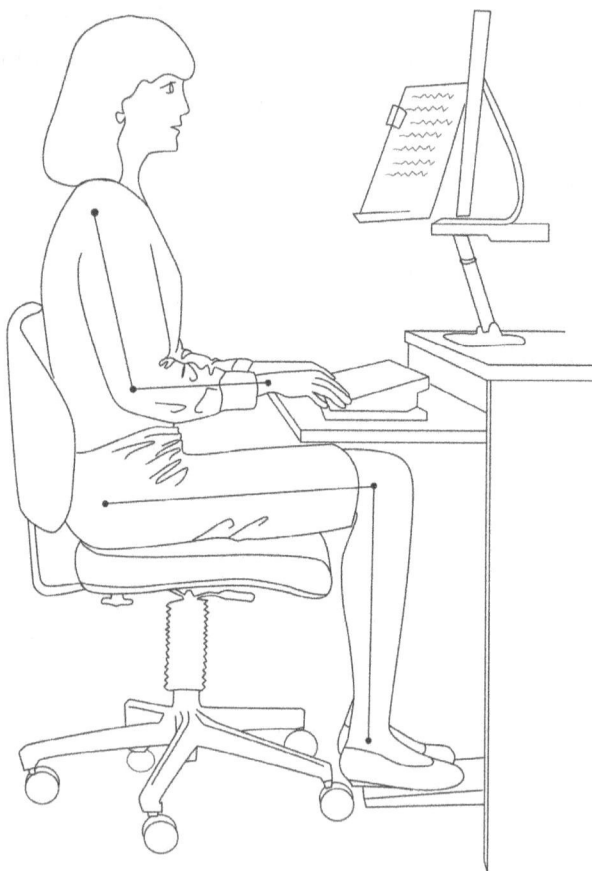

Let's build from this base.

Now you are sitting in front of your computer at a desk with a keyboard shelf and a big screen monitor.

1. Your arms are hanging at your sides. Bend at your elbows and bring your hands to rest at a 90° angle to your upper arm.

2. Raise or lower the chair so your hands rest on the keyboard, hands slightly lower than your elbows.

3. A good angle for your thighs would be for your knees to be slightly higher than your pelvis or at a 90° angle from your pelvis. If you need to, put something under your feet to raise your thighs off the chair relieving any pull on your pelvis, low back and compression on the backs of the thighs. If the desk from above is compressing your thighs, tilt the seat downward giving your thighs more room. Recheck all adjustments often.

4. The top of the monitor should be at about your eye level.

5. Your chest is lifted and open. Relax between the front of your shoulders.

Sitting at any workstation is hard on your body. Think of it as a fluid-filled position like a bowl of water - always changing and seeking balance.

TOUCHING YOU with words

What I have learned

and know to be true is

"People want to learn about their bodies!"

Take notes about the pain you feel.

_____

_____

_____

_____

_____

_____

_____

_____

Pain Management is: Awareness, Relief, Prevention

_____

_____

_____

_____

_____

_____

_____

_____

*Additional tools at **www.TouchOfMary.com***
We Have Tutorial Videos

CHAPTER 3

Standing

ASK   **TAKE INVENTORY**   *WHAT AM I DOING?*

LISTEN   **EVALUATE**   *HOW IS THIS AFFECTING ME?*

RESPOND   **MAKE CHANGE**   *WHAT CAN I DO DIFFERENTLY?*

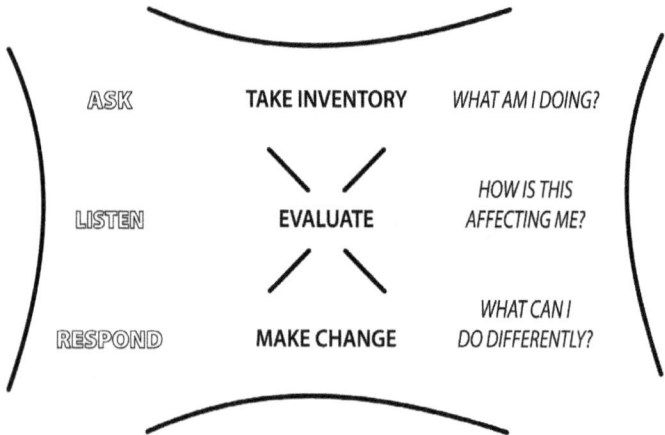

Act: as if it is the first time you are taking inventory every time you take inventory!

You: will be open to new information with this approach.

*Additional tools at **www.TouchOfMary.com***

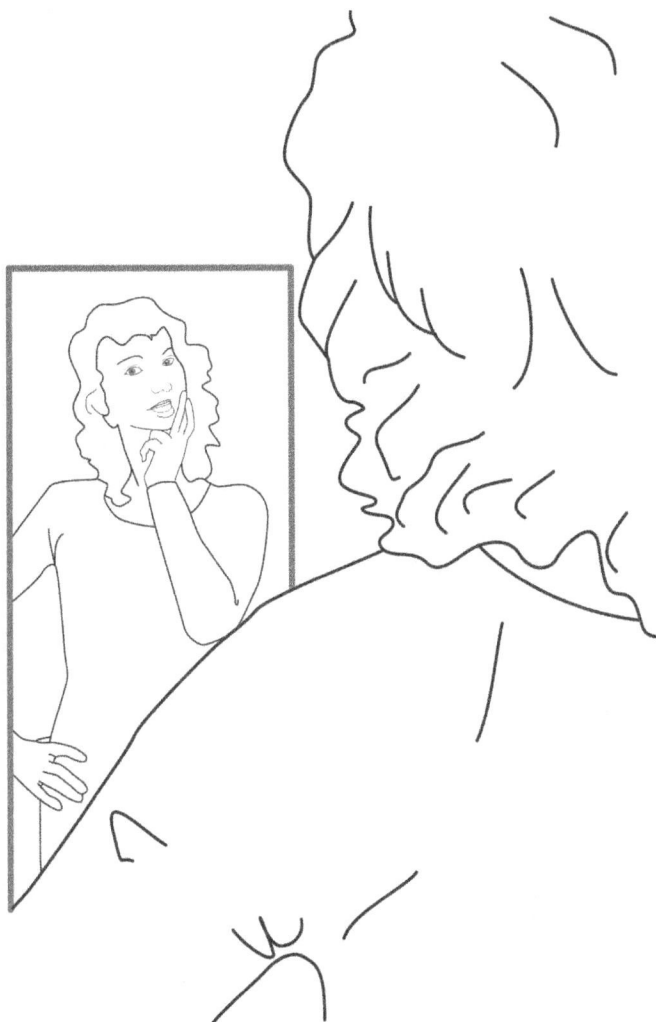

What do I notice?

Standing

Standing is so simple, or is it?

Are you aware of how you are doing this thing called standing?

Let's start our query here.

Stand flatfooted; feet shoulder width apart, pelvis relaxed, spine straight, eyes looking at the horizon. Look at yourself in front of a full-length mirror or have someone give you feed back about what they see.

Ask yourself these questions:

1. Are my feet side by side facing forward or is one foot in front of the other and angled out to the side?

2. Is one hip kicked out to the side?

3. What about the shoulders - are they level?

4. Look at your face in the mirror. Is the chin jutted out to the side or tucked into the chest?

5. Scan your body and notice whatever you can. Close your eyes and feel what it is like to be in your body right now.

Let's gain more information and explore how to change what is happening.

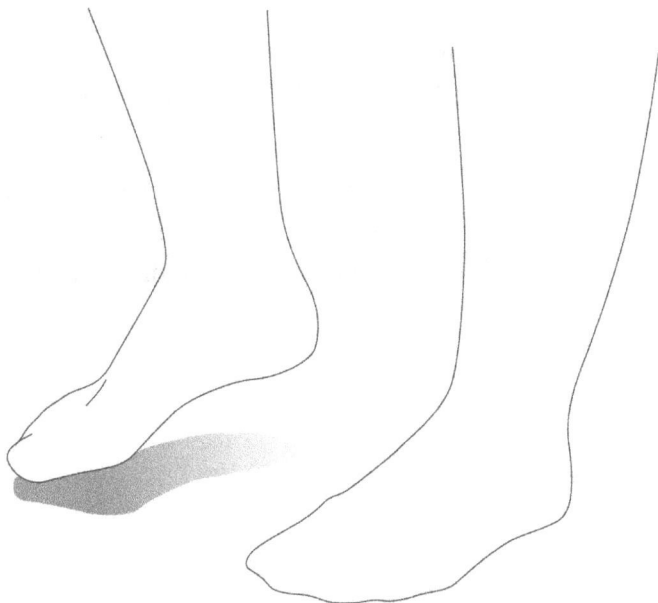

Exercise: *Shift your weight one foot to the other foot several times as you lift one foot off the ground. Feeling 100% of your weight transfer to the hip, down the leg into the foot being stood upon.*

Let's Experiment.

1. Shift your weight from one foot to the other, picking up one foot. Do not lift the foot high – just enough so all of your weight is on one foot.

2. Now shift your weight to the other foot, lifting the opposite foot off the ground. Repeat (1 & 2) until you get the feel of your weight completely shifting from side to side.

3. Now stop and feel where you land in your feet – is it the same as when you started? Where is your weight in your feet? Equal in both or more on one side than the other?

4. Where in your feet is the weight placed? Forward in the toes or back in the heels or even to the outside / inside? One foot may be different than the other.

5. Check in at the knees. Are they locked back or not?

6. Move your awareness up to the hips. Shift your hips from side to side. What do you feel in your feet? Is the weight shifting between your feet?

7. Move now to the rib cage. Shift your rib cage from side to side. Then twist your rib cage one direction then the other. What do you feel in your feet? Is the weight shifting between your feet?

8. Now move your awareness to the shoulders. Move the shoulders up and down, together and then one at a time. Again what is happening in your feet?

Repeat steps #4 through #8 above with one foot in front of the other. Now reverse your feet and repeat. Notice how this affects your weight distribution between the feet and what is different about moving the upper body.

The position of every body part (including your feet) can effect how you are standing.

If you have any pain standing, go through this exercise and choose a different standing position. Always find your center first and adjust from there to find a less painful position.

This exercise will also give you feedback about what might be tight and need to be stretched, or what is weak and needs to be strengthened.

And shoes throw in a whole new element. Try this exercise with different shoes on and notice what changes.

Did you ever think there could be so much involved in STANDING?

> *More Insight:* High heels can force the body into a strained posture. Opening and lengthening at the closed joints is the way to relieve the strain caused by wearing heels. See illustrations on pages 28 & 29.

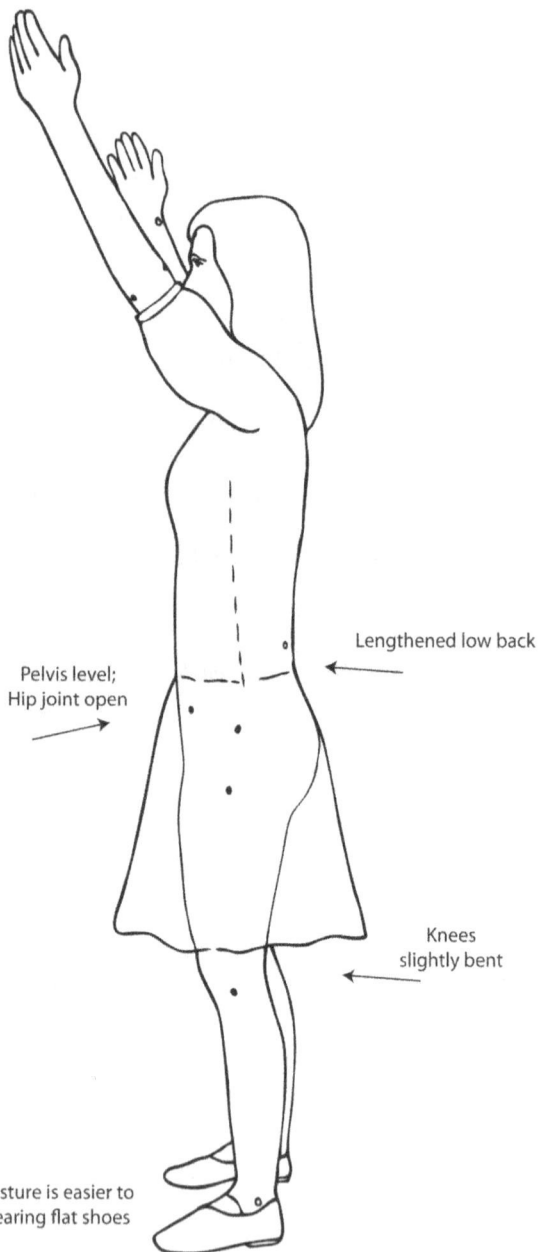

Lengthened low back

Pelvis level;
Hip joint open

Knees
slightly bent

This body posture is easier to
maintain wearing flat shoes

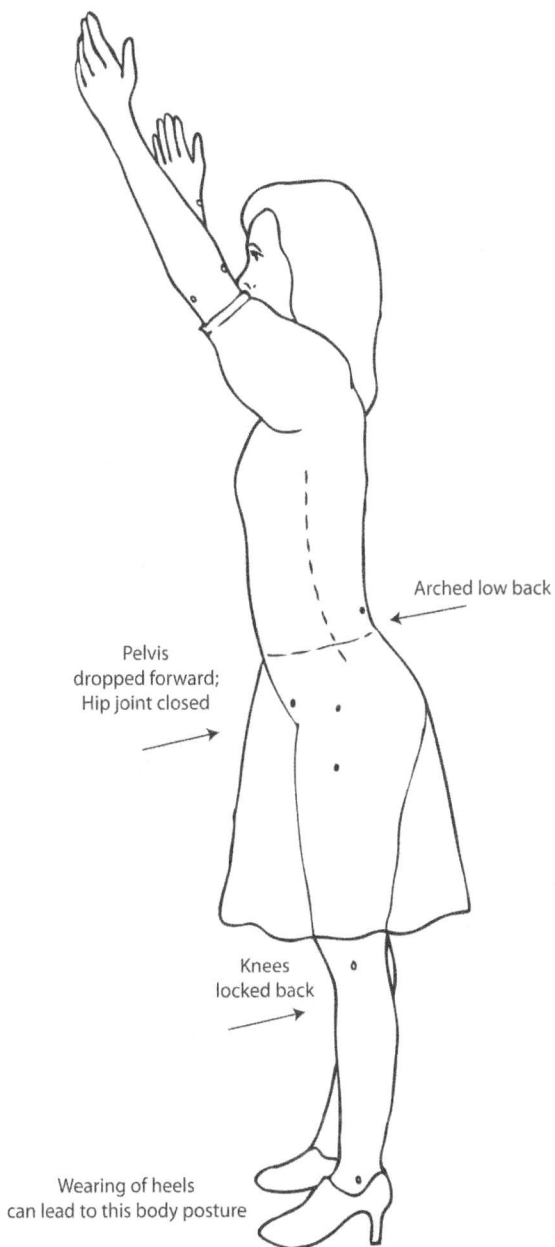

Arched low back

Pelvis
dropped forward;
Hip joint closed

Knees
locked back

Wearing of heels
can lead to this body posture

TOUCHING YOU with words

"As a child you learn to move through mimicry.

Watching those around you, mom, dad, brother, sister, etc...

and then coping what you observe."

Take notes about when you feel the pain eases or it goes away. What were you doing?

_____

_____

_____

_____

_____

_____

_____

_____

Pain Management is: Awareness, Relief, Prevention

_____

_____

_____

_____

_____

_____

_____

*Additional tools at **www.TouchOfMary.com***
We Have Tutorial Videos

CHAPTER 4

Walking

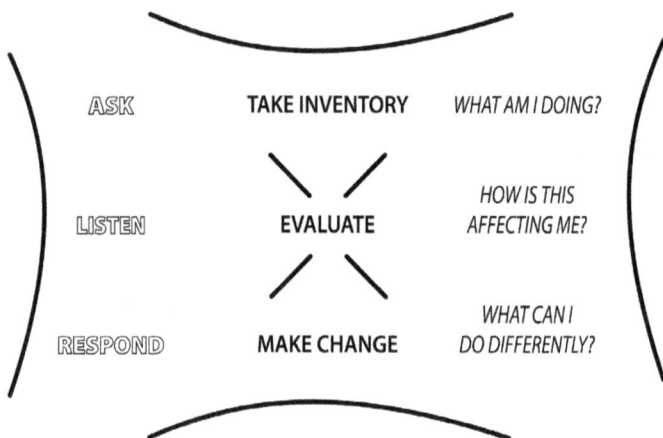

ASK	TAKE INVENTORY	WHAT AM I DOING?
LISTEN	EVALUATE	HOW IS THIS AFFECTING ME?
RESPOND	MAKE CHANGE	WHAT CAN I DO DIFFERENTLY?

Act: as if it is the first time you are taking inventory every time you take inventory!

You: will be open to new information with this approach.

*Additional tools at **www.TouchOfMary.com***

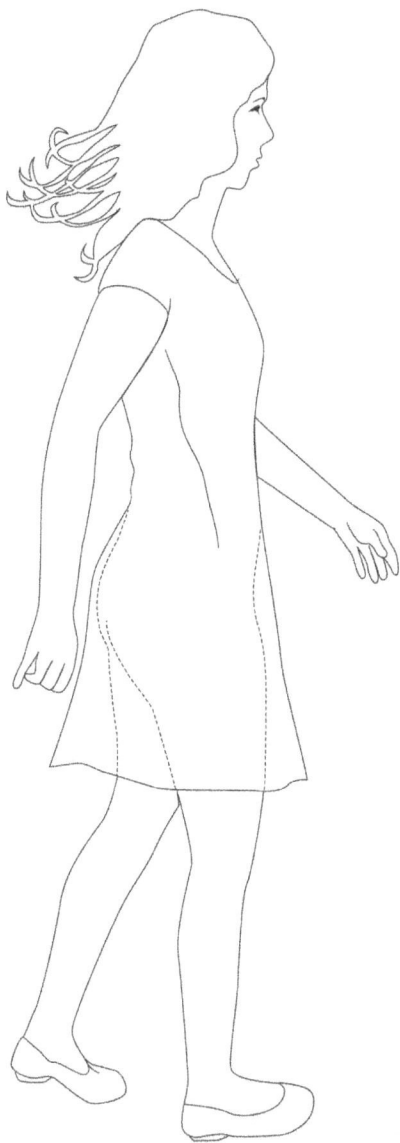

Walking

Now that you are standing with more awareness of your placement in space, let's start to propel ourselves forward.

Start walking in a line or big circle on flat ground. Around the block or up and down the driveway or even a long hallway will work. Begin to notice how you are moving through space.

Ask yourself these questions:

- Are my kneecaps pointed in the direction I am going?

- Are both of my arms swinging?

- Are they moving forward and backward equally (shoulders and elbow movement)?

- Are my arms swinging opposite of my legs? At this point adjust arm movements if needed.

- Are my ribs moving or are they feeling stuck?

- Let your ribs move with the arms, rotating the ribs opposite of the hips and feet.

- What is happening to the spine? Is it stiff? Can you feel or tell?

The spine will have to twist for the ribs to move and the torso to rotate opposite of the hips. Also twisting the spine will make you stand up taller and straighter. Just the biomechanics of the bones at work here.

Are these movements hard or easy to do? Sometimes there is a coordination issue and practice *will* help.

Continue walking, noticing more things like:

What are my feet doing as I walk?

How do I strike the ground with each foot and then roll off the toes?

Are both feet doing the same thing?

This is how the legs, knees and feet should work together for walking:

- With the <u>kneecap</u> pointing in the direction you intend to go. Bend the leg at the hip with the knee, swinging the <u>thigh</u> forward, letting the leg movement pull and roll the foot off the ground.

- Strike the ground gently with the heel.

- Next the little toe then big toe land on the ground.

- Leave the ground the same way allowing the <u>thigh swing</u> to pull the heel off the ground.

- Then the little toe and big toe follow. Relax and open the ankle.

- You may not perceive the separate parts. This all happens very quickly. Strive for a fluid motion.

Addition note: *Focusing on the **thigh swing** and the **direction that the kneecap is pointed in** is the most important part. Allow the foot to land as best it can.*

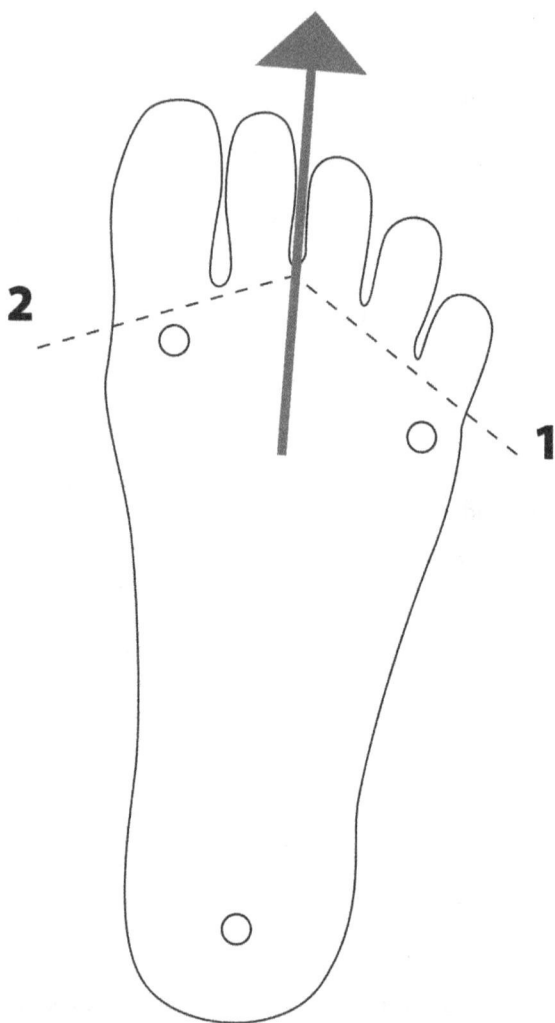

Other places in the body to look for variances are:

- **Knees:** Are they locking back or is one knee locking and the other not?

- **Hips:** Are they both moving up and down the same amount?

- **Posture:** Am I leaning forward or backward with my head or chest?

The notion that the body can be in a perfect alignment is, in my opinion, a misconception. I believe the body only passes through this (central) perfect alignment as it adapts its form to accomplish the next function.

TOUCHING YOU with words

"You are the only one with you

24/7

so who better to ask than you?"

Take note about your sleeping position.

_____

_____

_____

_____

_____

_____

_____

_____

Pain Management is: Awareness, Relief, Prevention

_____

_____

_____

_____

_____

_____

_____

_____

*Additional tools at **www.TouchOfMary.com***
We Have Tutorial Videos

Lying Down

ASK **TAKE INVENTORY** *WHAT AM I DOING?*

LISTEN **EVALUATE** *HOW IS THIS AFFECTING ME?*

RESPOND **MAKE CHANGE** *WHAT CAN I DO DIFFERENTLY?*

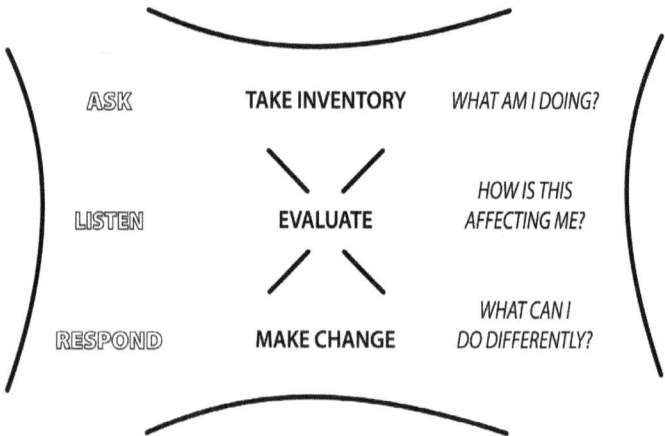

Act: as if it is the first time you are taking inventory every time you take inventory!

You: will be open to new information with this approach.

*Additional tools at **www.TouchOfMary.com***

Lying Down

Lying down: what a great thing to do!

- Where do you lie down? On the floor, couch or bed?

- What position? On your back, side or stomach?

- Are you reading, watching TV, resting, sleeping or on the computer?

- How much support do you receive from the furniture or floor?

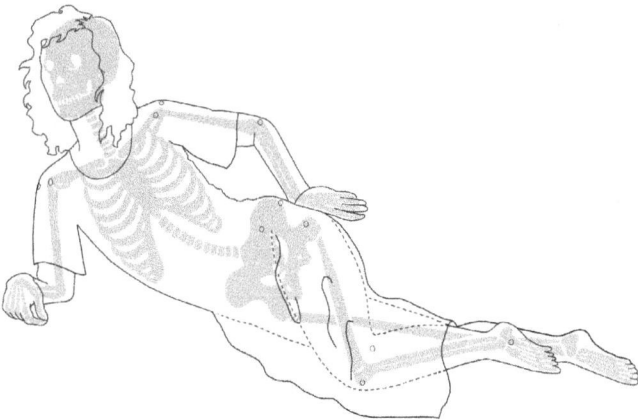

How long can you lie in this position and be comfortable?

We will discuss the bed and sleeping here but you can use the same information for other activities.

We all have different preferences when it comes to furniture but the bed where we sleep is of the greatest importance to most of us. A good night's sleep is wonderful!

If your body is flexible and the joints open and adjust easily you can take (and usually like) a firmer surface. A very soft surface offers little support and can require the joints to grab / cling together to hold you up.

If your body is more locked in one or more areas a softer surface is required to let those body parts have their way (staying in a fixed position).

I believe if you are tossing all night, it is due to your body being uncomfortable and asking you to move - like squirming in a chair when you are uncomfortable.

Stand up and place your body in the position that you sleep in and see how long you can hold that position. You are spending many hours in this position at night when sleeping. Now can you begin to understand why you may hurt in the morning?

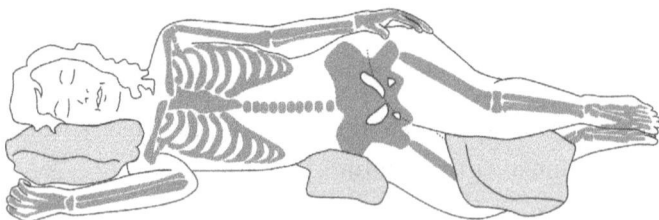

Let's go back to what position you like to sleep in. Is it on your stomach, on your back or on your side? It could be some kind of half position of side and stomach combined.

The stomach position is not a good one to sleep in and if you have this habit please do break yourself of it. Your back and neck will be forever grateful!

If you sleep on your side

Keep the spine level or straight. At the neck fill the L shape area between the shoulder and head to keep the spine in alignment.

Next use a big pillow or teddy bear to wrap your arms around - to keep your arms from becoming folded like chicken wings or tucked under your head. This will help the shoulders stay open.

Next where are you knees and feet? If one knee is in front of the other and both knees are resting on the bed your hips will be twisted. This twisting can irritate the low back and more. Use a pillow to stack them on top of each other. A long body pillow could be useful here and make turning a bit easier.

Lying on your back

Something under your knees will make it easier on a stiff low back.

Keep the pillow under your head to a minimum thickness or just put a small roll under your neck.

Note: *If your shoulders tend to be rounded forward, lying on your back can leave them hanging in mid air causing pain and numbness. A folded pillowcase tucked under you at the top of each of the shoulder blades, lifting and holding them off the bed surface, can help.*

If you start on your back and then roll to the side notice which moves first the head or the feet, knees or hips? You can block this area in place with pillows to keep from rolling onto your side.

Changing sleeping patterns requires commitment. If you have a partner who sleeps in your bed, ask them to wake you if they see you in a position you want to avoid.

All that you do adds up to how your body arrives at having pain.

_____

_____

_____

_____

_____

_____

_____

_____

Pain Management is: Awareness, Relief, Prevention

_____

_____

_____

_____

_____

_____

_____

*Additional tools at **www.TouchOfMary.com***
We Have Tutorial Videos

CHAPTER 6

System of Change

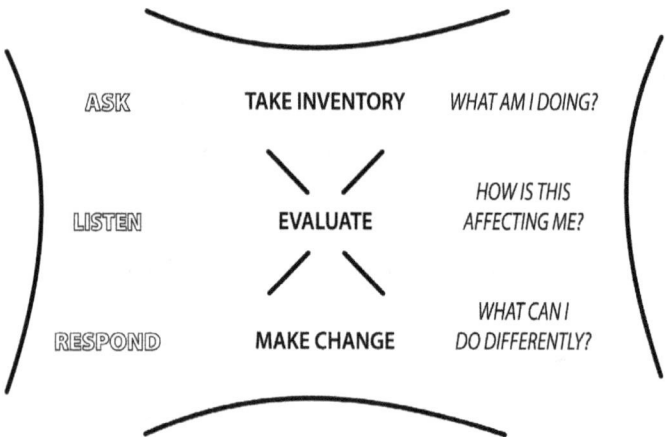

ASK   TAKE INVENTORY   WHAT AM I DOING?

LISTEN   EVALUATE   HOW IS THIS
AFFECTING ME?

RESPOND   MAKE CHANGE   WHAT CAN I
DO DIFFERENTLY?

Act: as if it is the first time you are taking inventory every time you take inventory!

You: will be open to new information with this approach.

*Additional tools at **www.TouchOfMary.com***

A rusty old car that has run down the road for 30 years with one oversized wheel rim works just fine till someone goes and puts the correct size wheel rim on. Oh! What a creaky, achy chunk of metal.

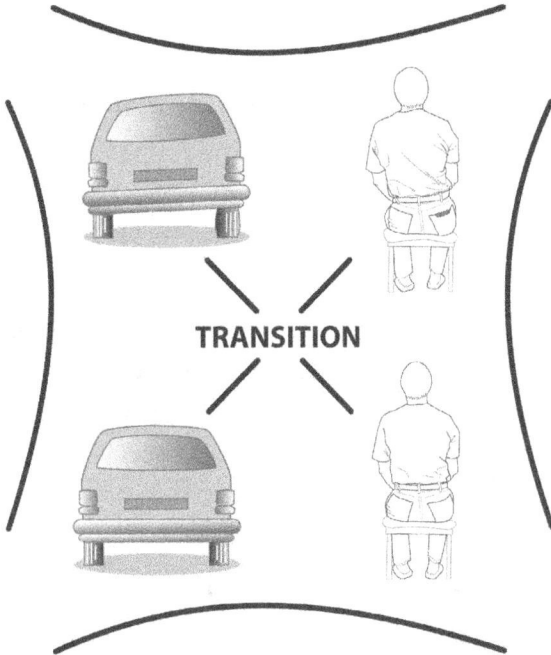

TRANSITION

The same thing happens when a person holds unbalanced patterns in the body. Like sitting on a wallet kept in the back hip pocket day after day. Oops! Now the wallet is elsewhere.

There will be a transition period.

System of Change

The body is built to adapt and it has a priority list of body parts and systems that are protected first. I think this list varies from person to person.

The body becomes fixated for many reasons: adhesions in the fascia, scars in the soft tissue, or breaking or misplacement of the bones (due to holding and use patterns). Then the body will adapt to make these fixations functional within your body. (Fixations are very tightly held body positions). You will find a fixated (tightly held) area above and below an area that is unstable (loosely held).

When the body has adapted to its limit the fixations can change. A small thing like bending over can strain something in the body depending on your particular adaptation and fixation pattern. A car accident can break one or many fixations and totally change how the system (your body) works together (not fun)!

Your body can have fixations in a few areas and can be very functional. It's when these functional fixations break that pain can be very hard to ignore and even harder to work through in order to regain the previous level of function.

The breaking loose of tissues holding onto a fixation (posture) pattern can be very painful.

1. The tissues have to calm down.

2. Then they need to be stretched and then strengthened.

3. And finally you must build new muscle memory to hold the new (improved) pattern.

This is a cycle.

> *A transition can be one or more cycles of release and stabilization.*

Prevention is the best option. Listen when the pain speaks up and change what you are doing.

1. Keep The System Flexible.

2. Develop Your Listening & Evaluation Skills.

3. Change Your Behavior When Pain Directs You To.

Gentle stretching of the whole body (forward / backward / side-to-side / twisting in both directions) will keep the fascia (or elastic) flexible, therefore making adaptation (change) easier.

> *This will not fix everything but it will take you down a very rewarding path.*
>
> *Form follows function.*
> *Function follows form.*
> *They are interdependent.*

In closing, I want to suggest a way to incorporate new habits of caring for your body that anyone can find the time for.

1. Choose five simple stretching exercises.

2. Do one each day prior to going to bed (3 minutes max.)

3. Rotate through the 5 stretches, doing a different one each day. If you have gone to bed and not done your one exercise *get back up and do it.*

4. By the end of the week you will have done 7 stretches and spent less than 30 min. total!

This is how to establish a new habit. And if your body feels better for doing it, the time *may* magically expand.

And most important of all, your body will have felt heard.

Acknowledgments

I would like to express my deepest gratitude to my mentors, instructors, students and clients who exposed me to their knowledge and brought me their bodies' pain, looking for answers. Their questions always brought me a deeper understanding of myself - as I did my best to provide assistance. I believe the real healer is within.

I would also like to thank Nicki Connors for listening to her inner voice to help pick the title of this book.

Russ Whitney, thank you! Without your encouragement I would have stopped three feet from gold.

Mark Paul your advice has been invaluable. Thanks!

Linda Ouellet I truly needed your help with the French translation. Merci beaucoup!

And Christine Lorenz you are a treasured friend of mine.

Praise for "Hello! This is your body speaking."

Foremost

It is evident immediately what is evoked with simplicity. The drawings redouble the impact. The mind will look to its internal process, trying to shorten the path, just to satisfy its own ideas. *With simplicity, this is unnecessary.* The educational objective is to create everything from where memory already lives.

The little book that Mary offers responds perfectly to this mental journey: that the essence of our movements, when done well, can guide us though our daily activities. Simply reading it and looking at the drawings will produce the desired impact. If we are open-minded and receptive to it, the goal is already achieved.

Who doesn't openly embrace simplicity?

It is very pleasing to me to see a major shortcut established by one of my students – after having spent a good part of my life sharing my professional experience in the domain of movement with awareness. And to observe that with time what we share bears fruit, and then tirelessly continues to progress on its own path, shaped by the personality who has received it.

Mary, my best wishes accompany you on this path that opens before you. -*Alain Géhin, D.O., Barcelona, February 2012*

Forward

From the moment I heard the title of this book, I knew it was a book that needed to be read..by lots of people. As a massage therapist for over 35 years, I have experienced many times – with my clients and myself - that our bodies are trying desperately to have a conversation with us. But it seems that we mostly listen to them when they are shouting.

Mary Wheeler is one of those rare people who "listens" to bodies with her heart, mind, hands, intuition, and even her eyes. She is a structural engineer masquerading as a massage therapist because she can discern the structural strengths and weaknesses people carry in their bodies – some hidden and some visible - that others might miss.

That she wrote this book and shared some of her observations and talents is wonderful. That she writes about it in a way that is easily readable and accessible to learn is amazing.

I am honored to introduce you to this book. But most of all I am excited to share this secret: we would all do well – therapists and lay people alike – to start listening when our bodies are whispering, talking, and yes even shouting. It is never too late to begin the conversation. - *Christine Lorenz, B.A., LMT*

Endorsements

"Reading this book requires a leap of faith - as you look at your body from a different perspective. You will be glad you did. It clearly lays out how to better understand what your body is telling you - and what to do about it. In fact, with just a few minutes a day, you can start down the path to a healthier lifestyle." *-Mark Paul, Managing Partner at Synergy Consulting Group and author: of "The Entrepreneur's Survival Guide", "How to Attract Significantly More Customers" and "The 21st Century Energy Initiative: How to Solve our Energy Problems."*

"In Hello! This is your body speaking- Is anyone listening?" Mary Wheeler artfully presents a simple, easy to understand guide of proactive methods to "listen" and react when your body is speaking. She has successfully bridged the act of personally coaching you (being there) to guiding you through a written workbook.

As a pharmacist with many patients suffering from chronic pain, I often wish I had an easier way to refer them to someone of Ms. Wheeler's caliber. This workbook, with chapters on the biomechanics of sitting, standing, and lying down serves as a wonderful introduction to what Ms. Wheeler teaches on how to "be-friend my pain." Its pages are full of insightful, wonderfully illustrated advice on how to take self-inventory, evaluate, and finally make changes that lead to a healthier, happy life.

My earnest wish is that my patients and many others use this book, and learn from Ms. Wheeler's many years of successful therapy that she has graciously shared with us."
-Kathryn L Hahn, PharmD, DAAPM, CPE / Pharmacy Manager, Bi-Mart Corp. / Chair, Oregon Pain Management Commission / Affiliate Faculty, Oregon State University College of Pharmacy.

"Mary Wheeler's book "Hello! This is your body speaking to you-Is anyone listening?" has captured a realistic way of checking in with your "self." The pains that could be attributed to everyday life is just that, pains of everyday life! Learning to pay attention to how you use your self when you are moving, sitting, and standing can make everyday life a wonderful experience! Taking the time to experience the positives and not so positive feelings are expressed in her material with great pictures of the body moving thru space, and also with the body being still! Mary has found a way to put together a great self checklist for the reader and the mover! Open your mind and listen to your body, so you can enjoy yourself!"
-Denise Thomas-Morrow / Fitness Specialist / Certified Alexander Technique Teacher / Owner of Let's Move Fitness, Alignment and Dance Studio

Testimonials from Mary's Clients

"Mary helps me "take a step forward" in dealing with pain and other physical challenges. She teaches me how to interpret signals from my body so that I can be an active participant in addressing problems that had prevented me from participating in the activities I enjoy.

Mary provides me with goals to work toward, gets me started in the right direction, and the means for me to make progress on my own.

Mary finds root causes of pain." -Lynn Coody, Organic Agsystems Consulting, Eugene, OR

"Mary has been my exclusive massage therapist, treating me on a regular schedule for years. Her professionalism has always been of the utmost quality. At each visits she gives me a detailed examination of what new problem might need special attention and what behavior or condition might have caused it. She also reviews what had been problematic at the last session in case that still needs some work. Lastly she will always take time to teach me stretching, walking modifications, or any other therapeutic recommendations that might help improve my physical movements." *-Daniel Delsman, Dan Delsman Painting Co., Eugene, OR*

About the Author

Mary Wheeler lives in Eugene, Oregon and has been a Massage Therapist since 1993. She specializes in movement analysis and does medical massage. This book is only the tip of the iceberg in a small location on a vast map. Mary loves to dance, sew, walk, read and watch movies on the silver screen.

*Contact her at: **www.TouchOfMary.com***

Resources

These are many of the resources I have used through out my lifetime. Which have all helped me to accomplish the writing and publishing of this book as well as maintain a healthy body.

- A Course In Miracles: acim.org

- Anatomy of the Spirit: Caroline Myss, Ph.D.

- Atlas of Manipulative Techniques for the Cranium & Face: Alain Géhin

- Awakening Intuition: Dr. Mona Lisa Schulz

- Cash Flow Game: www.richdad.com

- Cross-Crawl Exercises: Google it.

- Deep Tissues Sculpting: Carole Osborne-Sheets

- Denise Thomas-Morrow: Let's Move Fitness Studio www.letsmovewithd.com

- Detoxify or Die: Sherry A. Rogers, M.D.

- DJ Launch Academy: www.djlaunchacademy.com

- Eat Right 4 Your Type: Peter J. D'Adamo & Catherine Whitney

- Energy Medicine: James L. Oschman

- Facial Yoga: www.starface.com

- German New Medicine: www.newmedicine.ca

- Heal Your Body: Louise Hay

- Healing Massage: Techniques: Frances M. Tappan

- Inner Voice: Russ Whitney

- Intuitive Healing: Dr. Judith Orloff

- Mary Wheeler: www.TouchOfMary.com

- Molecules of Emotion: Candace B. Pert

- Multiple Sclerosis: Judy Graham

- Outwitting the Devil:
  www.outwittingthedevil.com

- Pain Society of Oregon: www.painsociety.com

- Prolotherapy: www.getprolo.com

- Rich Dad Poor Dad: Robert Kiyosaki

- Semi-Supine: Alexander Technique

- Strengths Based Leadership:
  www.gallupstrengthscenter.com

- The Anatomy Coloring Book: Kapit / Elson

- The Entrepreneur's Survival Guide: Mark Paul
  www.synergyusa.com

- The Influencer:
  www.youtube.com/watch?v=l4g_xxguWzI

- The Price of Everything: Eduardo Porter

- The Vortex: Esther and Jerry Hicks

- Think and Grow Rich: Napoleon Hill

- Wilson's Temperature Syndrome:
  www.wilsonssyndrome.com